I0436986

It's All HAIR

It's All HAIR

Healthy • Acceptance • Inspiring • Reality

Detrice Milliner-Sims

Copyright © 2012 by Detrice Milliner-Sims.

ISBN:	Softcover	978-1-4797-2750-6
	Ebook	978-1-4797-2751-3

All rights reserved. No part of this book may be reproduced or transmitted in any form or by any means, electronic or mechanical, including photocopying, recording, or by any information storage and retrieval system, without permission in writing from the copyright owner.

This book was created in the United States of America.

To order additional copies of this book, contact:
Xlibris Corporation
1-888-795-4274
www.Xlibris.com
Orders@Xlibris.com
122344

Contents

Section 2

I wish to say, "Thank you" to all hair professionals that have worked with me over the years. I also wish to say, "Thank you" to all my clients who have supported me and shared their most intimate thoughts with me; some of tears, others of laughter. I would like to express my gratitude to those difficult clients I have had who have helped me build character. Of course, I would like to thank my friends and family who were always so patient and understanding with me. And finally, but certainly not least, I would like to give a special thanks to my husband for all the hard work he did behind the scene.

Above all, I wish to say, "Thank you my Creator, for the knowledge and wisdom you have given me to guide my life."

CONSULTATION AND YOUR HAIR

Healthy hair starts with a trusted professional consultation. It is important to know and understand your hair type. If what the professional says does not make sense, find another. The only separation of a hair professional is the education they received, coupled with good sense and honesty. If what you hear and what you see or what you know does not make sense about your hair, try another consultation. This includes being an honest client. If you are not honest, your hair will not be honest to you.

SHAMPOOING AND CONDITIONING YOUR HAIR

There is one major factor to the variety of culture and their hair. It is its cleansing power. This could be done daily, weekly or bi-weekly. Allowing one's hair to go unclean for long periods of time invites fungus or bacteria or possible hair loss (When this occurs, it is recommended that one seek the help of a licensed physician). This can result in damaging your hair and an unhealthy hair condition.

For healthy hair, it is the cleansing power that works. Choosing one or more shampoos and conditioners is best. Just as eating the same foods become boring to us, so is using the same shampoo and conditioner. Hair wants a different menu of food from time to time. Select a variety suitable to your hair type. Switch to the response of your hair behavior. Shampoo and conditioner of the same product line works best. It softens the hair and makes it manageable, attractive, touchable, beautiful and shiny. Avoid using conditioners that only coat the hair. These leave hair heavy or flat. Moisturizing conditioner penetrates the hair and can be used daily. Deep conditioners are also penetrating and can be used weekly combined with a hot oil treatment. This helps to invigorate the hair. Over-conditioning can leave hair the limp and lifeless. It is best to follow the directions given for proper use. A hair texture that varies in type may require a combination of conditioners. Some have that exotic hair, highly different in texture.

CUTTING YOUR HAIR

This is often a huge problem to having healthy hair. It is important to have haircuts. It is recommended on the average to have a half of an inch of hair cut every six weeks. Why so? It is like when you cut your toenails; it makes room for new nail growth. That toenail comes in strong and healthy. The toenail looks great (*not necessarily the toes*). Hair functions better when it is cut. Hair left uncut for long periods of time can lead to hair breakage (split ends) and hair loss. Don't let anyone fool you into thinking otherwise.

Some cultures cut children's hair as early as six months and this may vary. The same is true for them however. Children need their hair cut. Why not try what works best for your child, whether it is grandma, grandpa, mom or dad or a hair professional that is cutting the child's hair? These may be the most trusting for a child. The goal is to ensure healthy hair growth.

GLUE AND YOUR HAIR

Many use glue to add human or synthetic hair to their natural hair. This form of hair extension has proved damaging to hair. The truth of the matter is glue inhibits the naturalness of your hair and its oils and because of this, many people over-use it. This should never be a permanent solution to hair care. Its results are damaging and extremely uncomfortable and in some cases, hair loss is irreversible.

If you use glue for hair extensions, it should only be done for special occasions with the thought of removing it in a few days. Always use a hair solution that allows the hair to separate from its foundation without snapping or breaking the hair or causing irritation to the hair scalp. Look good, wear it well, but remember to remove it soon. It is always better to have a healthy head of hair to work with when desiring to enhance your beauty.

HAIR WEAVES AND YOUR HAIR

This form of hair extension is very popular today. The natural hair is braided or twisted and human hair or synthetic hair is sewed to it. This has some advantages over gluing the hair, but there are some disadvantages.

When hair is permed, relaxed, colored or bleached it is in a fragile state. Weaving in hair extensions too soon often results in hair breakage. Sewing hair in too tightly causes breakage and when removing it improperly can cause damage. I have seen some clients cut patches out of their hair. Just like it takes time to sew it in, it takes time to remove it. It's like a hem to a dress; if you remove it properly, the material remains in tack. Remove your hair weaves properly by taking your time to cut each threaded stitch. Pull the hair gently as it loosens.

Many who use hair weaving extensions don't provide themselves with proper hair care. Shampooing and conditioning the hair is highly important for your own hair to remain healthy. Try this method, part your hair weave into four to six parts, softly braid each section, not pulling the hair too tightly and place a hair net over it. While in the shower, allow the water to run thru your hair. Next, place some shampoo in the palm of your hand and rub your fingertips in it and then gently message your scalp for a few minutes as you gently squeeze the rest of your hair. Rinse thoroughly. Do the same with the hair conditioner. This method prevents the hair from tangling. Gently blot the hair with a towel, removing excess water. Use a wide-tooth comb to clear the hair out. If needed you may then air dry or blow dry your hair, whichever works best for the type of hair you are wearing. Apply heat if you can, then style.

WIGS AND YOUR HAIR

"They have their places," said the wig wearer. Everyone should have a least one in their hair grooming collection for a "bad hair" day. This is the way to go. They come in all styles, shapes, sizes, and colors. They come as hair falls and ponytails. There are even have half hair wigs, short ones, long ones, expensive ones, and not so expensive ones. For the wig wearer, use it to enhance not to replace your hair.

Thinness comes with age. A health condition can make wearing a wig your only solution. Hair might grow in patches and this can be very uncomfortable to some. Many choose to cut their hair into one even length or wear a short sassy hairdo. Whatever suits your fancy; however, when wearing a wig, always give your hair "breaks" in-between. When in the privacy of your home, remove your wig and give your hair a chance to breath. Just as your skin needs sunlight, so does your hair.

Cutting your natural hair into a nice hairstyle can make you feel comfortable. This is inspiring to others when you are not using a wig. Young women, try to avoid wearing wigs as a permanent solution for your hair. Show your natural beauty. Don't lose it, wear it.

MEDICATION AND YOUR HAIR

Most people are on some kind of medication. These always have some adverse effect on your hair. Simply put, medication taken orally or intravenously, whether, legally or not, are chemicals that finds their way into the hair shaft. For those who take medication regularly, there are professional hair products that you can use to shampoo and condition your hair to help it to stay healthy. These products work to enhance the naturalness of your hair. The continued use of perms, relaxers, color and bleaches will eventually turn your hair to mush. The hair is left lifeless.

If possible, avoid using these chemicals when on medication. Semi-permanent and Demi-permanent colors also have chemical in them. Hair rinses works best because they don't have chemicals in it and it washes right out and can be used more frequently and are less damaging. The colors of the rainbow never changes and it is beautiful to see and so are we.

CHEMICALS AND YOUR HAIR

It is understood that all chemicals that are used to enhance the beauty of your hair is damaging or will cause damage to your hair when used for prolong periods. Yes, those chemical perms, relaxers, colors, and bleaches strip the hair of it naturalness. You look great, but remember, at some point in time, your hair is going to need a rest from these chemicals. Just as your body needs rest and refreshment, so does your natural hair.

Think of what your natural hair possess in it. Left without chemicals, it is always healthy, thicker and longer. Think about how you can utilize the natural oils in your hair to promote its healthiness. Acceptance and balance with proper hair care will lead to hair that's inspiring to others. Most of us have what we need; use it to show the reality of your hair.

HAIR TRANSPLANT AND YOUR HAIR

An innovating technique, hair transplant procedures, has become a solution for those who cannot deal with pre-mature baldness or hair loss of some kind. Men as well as women tend to prefer this form of hair extension because of its naturalness. One's own hair follicles are transplanted to an area of the head where baldness has occurred. I have cut the hair of many men who use this technique. The only drawback, they have told me, for most part was the pain they felt. We females know how men are when it comes to pain. So, you ladies be nice to them when they undergo this type of procedure and look beyond the obvious; they usually look good and younger in the end.

For the best results, a licensed physician should be consulted that specializes in the field of hair transplant. This is highly recommended, since it is a surgical procedure. More than one consultation will be wise before making a decision. Compare prices and know the history of the physician along with their star rating and use good judgment. The cost may vary in price. We only get what we pay for. Your goal should be a healthy hair transplant. Only then, will this make you feel good and that it was worth it.

COMB, BRUSHES AND HAIR EQUIPMENT FOR YOUR HAIR

For one's hair to maintain its healthiness, good sanitation of the hair equipment is essential. All hair equipment should be for personal use only. Every member of the household should have their personal hair grooming equipment. Using others' hair combs and brushes is a sure way to invite hair infections of some kind. Beware of professional hairstylist or barbers that do not sanitize their hair equipment after each use. It's like going to the doctor; if he doesn't wash his hands or wear protective gloves, please ask him to do so. If the appearance of the hair station and equipment is not sanitized, it is likely that the hair professional takes this too lightly and may lack good sanitation procedures. It's okay to remove yourself respectfully.

BRAIDING AND TWISTING YOUR HAIR

This has been around from the time we can remember. It's natural and healthier for your hair. Styles vary from culture to culture. Human or synthetic hair can be added to enhance hair attractiveness. Hair braiding can be used to return unhealthy hair and lost hair to its naturalness. It can be worn short or long. It is very widely accepted in some cultures when done with modesty.

Proper hair care is essential for a vibrant healthy look. Let your natural oils shine and use appropriate hair products. Avoid extreme styles that tend to distract from the natural beauty of your hair. When braiding the hair, avoid pulling it too tightly, as this prevents natural hair growth. It also causes headaches and hair breakage around the perimeter which can result in permanent hair loss (which is why there is no hair around your hair line.) It has been said that beauty is a pain. It doesn't have to be. The reality of it all is beauty should be comfortable. That's what makes you feel good within yourself.

SISTER LOCKS AND MICRO LOCKS AND YOUR HAIR

This has brought new awareness to culture and its hair. Many are opting for this natural look. "It makes me feel good about myself and my hair" and "No, more chemicals for me. It's my natural hair and I can wear it with dignity, style and keep it healthy," is what some clients have told me.

It is beautiful in its naturalness and can be worn with respect. There are a variety of hair styles that you can have. As you wear this style with modesty and neatness, you can inspire others to be comfortable with whom they are. Young and old love it. Seek a professional that is certified to perform this hair technique.

PRESS AND CURLING YOUR HAIR

There are many women wearing the long-lasting press and curl. Oh, what a task to do your hair, but it is healthy. Talk about self-esteem, this is a sure way to have it. Use small amount or hair wax or pressing oil on the hair only (AVOID PLACING IT ON THE SCALP).

When pressing your hair, use the back of the pressing comb to give your hair a straight look (AVOID GETTING TOO CLOSE TO THE SCALP). They make electric hot combs with temperature gauge so that you do not singe your hair. For a desired curl, use a curling iron. For a truly professional look, I recommend seeing a hair professional.

FLAT-IRONING YOUR HAIR

Flat-ironing the hair gives it a silky flow. This is the way to grace your hair and keep it healthy. Wear your natural hair between flat ironings to give it a rest from the heat of the iron. When doing it in the privacy of your home, shampoo your hair and use a deep conditioner mixed with hot oil. A dime or quarter size should be sufficient depending on the thickness and the length of your hair. Place a plastic cap over your hair and sit for fifteen minutes. Remove and rinse. This is a good way to lock in moisture. Next, blow dry. Section the hair into four or six parts and then, flat-iron by slicing your hair into small parts. Don't get too close to your scalp. As you flat-iron, pull the hair gently. Wrap your hair by parting it into four sections and comb the hair to flow in the direction you want it to go and wear a silk scarf before retiring to bed. This helps hold the style. Use an oil-sheen to enhance the hair.

HEALTHY SCALPS

Your scalp should show signs of healthiness. A healthy scalp is needed for healthy hair. If your scalp is healthy, your hair will be healthy, too. How often do you take time *just* to massage your scalp? Oiling or using hair pomade that is not too greasy or too heavy on your scalp is recommended for some cultures. Moderate amount of oil on the scalp and hair is not harmful. Place a small amount in the palm of your hand and gently massage with your fingertips. It helps promote good circulation for the scalp and prevent dryness. It looks vibrant and gives a healthy shine, which is attractive to others.

DON'T BE LAZY
ABOUT YOUR HAIR

Lacking the proper knowledge about hair care often leads to damaged hair. There are those who do not know how to care for their hair and those who fail to designate appropriate time for daily hair care. The result is unhealthy hair. Let's keep it real, there are people who devote more time to caring for their pet's hair then they do for their own hair. Laziness is not an option when it comes to good hair care. You can seek professional hair care and pay top dollar, but if you have a lazy attitude toward hair care, you will never be happy with yourself. If you don't have respect for your hair, others won't either. The more time you spend with other people, you get to know them well. The same is true with your hair. Spend time with it and you will get to know it well. It will treat you nicely.

FEED YOUR HAIR

What you eat will be reflected in your hair; healthy diet, healthy hair. As an infant grows in the mother's womb, so does its hair. When the infant is born, the hair is silky and shiny. Mothers giving birth to a newborn have a high self-awareness to a healthier diet; healthy diet, healthy newborn. The same is true for our hair. What we take into our bodies comes out in our hair. Learn to develop good healthy eating habits. Include vegetables and fruits, drink moderate amounts of water and don't forget to have a regular program of exercise. Good circulation is wonderful for healthy hair growth. The roots of your hair will be strong. Just as the body needs to be nourished and has hydration, with physical exercise, so does your hair.

CHILDREN'S HAIR

Children should be taught how to take proper care of their hair. Parents, this is a loving responsibility and aids in the bonding of you and your child. I always loved the way mom combed and brushed my hair. We teach our children how to say thank you, how to wash their hands and to respect each other. Yet, we spend little or no time teaching them how to care for their hair. Why not make it a part of your routine? When children's hair is left to chance, it can cause hair loss and breakage and various hair infections common to children such as hair lice, ringworms and other hair infections. These take months to clear up with the help of a licensed physician. This can be very devastating to a child. In some cultures, kids' hair left uncared for on a regular basis can become tangled and knotted. This may force the parent to cut the child's hair so that it can be manageable.

Kids want to be accepted by their peers, so educate them on how to care for their hair. Teach them how to grace their own natural hair. This helps them build character and self-respect. Young ones, wear it while you have it. Healthy hair means acceptance. Parents, remember your kids grow up to be adults.

SWIMMING IN THE POOL AND YOUR HAIR

Natural water does not cause damage to our hair. Water with chemicals does cause damage to our hair. Most swimming pools use a chlorine solution to sanitized the water and keep it safe for the swimmers. Hair chemicals and pool chemicals of any kind do not mix; it causes the hair to become dry and brittle. What happened to those swimming caps we use to wear. I don't know. But, if you find one and like its style, wear it. What I do know is if you are using chemical perms, relaxers, color and bleach on your hair, don't go swimming. If you love swimming, return to your natural hair. After having a fun day at the pool, shampoo and condition your hair. Use a deep conditioner or a hot old treatment that will help avoid dryness and breakage. Encourage other family members to do the same.

MEN AND THEIR HAIR

Generally, men show little interest in their hair. You see, they can attract a woman with or without hair. They do prefer women with hair. Hair care is just as important for them, so many of the same suggestions mentioned apply to them as well to promote healthy hair and healthy scalps. Men who are bald can purchase hair products to keep their scalp healthy. Men, use hair creams or oil that lock in moisture to prevent dryness. Most professional salons can provide what you need. Take the time to find out what works for you. Do you have those small hair sores on the nape of your head that keep multiplying and you can't seem to get rid of? The hair cutting equipment that is used on your hair may not be properly sanitized. Always, remember to request a shampoo and a skin antiseptic scalp conditioner after a haircut. See a licensed physician as he can determine the best treatment for that skin infection.

CLIMATE AND YOUR HAIR

From country to country, state to state, city to city, island to island, all hair types react differently to a climate change, sometimes for the good. It make sense if our mental, emotional and physical self has to make an adjustment when moving to a different climate; so does our hair. This could take months. Why not give your hair a helping hand and research your hair type before moving to your new horizon. This can allow your hair to make the transition and remain healthy. A different professional product line may be needed and this will help set it on the right path.

PRACTICAL, POSITIVE AND HELPFUL WAYS THAT BRING AWARENESS TO OUR HAIR IN CHANGING TIMES

THE "CURL" AND YOUR HAIR

Many women who have very thick coarse curly hair and many mature women desire to wear the curl; some remember it as the popular "Jeri Curl." It is easy to care for. This, too, is a very strong chemical and over a period of time, can cause hair loss. For other individuals, it works well because it allows their hair to remain moist. The professional hair product is design for use to moisturize and to help the hair to remain healthy. Don't get stuck in a rut when wearing the curl. Update your style get a nice professional haircut that will make it look fresh and sassy. Avoid permanent hair colors or bleaching. Double processing the hair can melt it away. Semi-permanent color or a rinse works best. Women's hair texture changes as she gets older. It becomes soft and manageable. It is wise to use a mild processing curl hair chemical for a change in texture or just let your own natural hair grow in while you enjoy those golden years. If you must use the Curl, seek out a licensed hair professional to perform this service. They have the knowledge needed for the best results. Wear your Curl gracefully and love who you are!!

GEL AND YOUR HAIR

Gel can be a useful product when enhancing the beauty of your hair. It can give your hair shine and hold. Beware of overuse. Gel that contains alcohol can dry the hair immensely. There are products that are alcohol-free so why not try these. Prolonged use can cause breakage and hair loss. If you must use a gel, try one that contains a hair moisturizer. You may want to combine a leave-in conditioner with you favorite gel. This locks in moisture. A non-flaking gel is recommended. This works well on curly and wavy hair. Mist the hair with a little water and use a wide tooth comb and brush gently with a soft bristle or just let your fingers flow through your hair. Let your natural curls define its style. Shampoo that cleanses the hair from build up is preferable, along with a deep conditioner and a hot oil treatments on a weekly basis. Your hair will grow as it remains healthy.

SPRAYING AND SPRITZING YOUR HAIR

Some desire to hold their hairstyle in place with spraying and spritzing products. These products may contain alcohol. Again, try searching out products that are alcohol-free, to prevent your hair from becoming too dry. Hair pump bottles verses spray cans are better for those who suffer with allergies. Many over use these products. The result is the hair becomes dry and brittle with much build up. In some cases, you can actually see the build up of hairspray. When using these products, avoid getting too close to the hair. Hold the product above or away and spray-mist the hair while styling. Shampoo that cleanses the hair from build up is recommended. Deep conditioner with hot oil treatments, done weekly, help hair to remain soft and manageable.

FIVE DOLLAR HAIRCUT OR
A FIFTY DOLLAR HAIRCUT

What is the difference? The hairstylist that is cutting your hair is what makes the difference. The price you pay is your preference, but remember, there are very good hairstylists that have an outstanding ability to cut hair no matter what the price. Many people are feeling the pinch these day so when adjusting your budget, look for a hairstylist that can give you that professional cut you want. Try this when entering a salon: Sit and observer the hairstylist. Watch out for those hairstylists who cut hair without parting or sectioning the hair. A good professional hair cutter always sections the hair before cutting. They have a starting point and a finishing point. Blending the cut is important to them. The hair falls in all the right places and it is even and well arranged. Clipper cuts may differ slightly but there should be a starting and ending point. There are hair textures (curly) that cuts well with a razor. Wetting the hair gives a better razor cut to the hair. When you find a professional that gives good razor cuts, stick with that professional. When visiting a salon, respectfully approach the hairstylist and converse with the professional. This should help you feel confident that the hairstylist can give you the desired cut you are requesting.

RELAXING, COLORING, AND BLEACHING CHILDREN HAIR

This is a question that has been posed to me many, many times in the business, "Should I relax, color or bleach my child's hair." This is a personal decision that parents need to decide. Let me give you some food for thought. When choosing to put these strong chemicals in a minor child's hair consider that these chemicals are damaging to the hair. If these chemicals are damaging to an adult's hair, especially when used for a prolong periods of time, what do you think it will do to a child's hair? The hair is an appendage of the skin and if a chemical can burn the skin, what will it do to the child's scalp? They are just too young and lack the responsibility for proper care. They are still maturing into young adults and time is needed to allow the hormones to move around (and any parent who has raised children knows what those hormones can do when those hormones start moving around!). Your child may look nice and feel good among their peers, but unless you as the parent is willing to face the *task* of caring for the child's hair, think twice. Teach the child to grace her own natural hair and how to care for it. When the child reaches the age of responsibility, enough to care for the hair with a chemical, have the child go to a professional to start the process properly. If the child has learn how to provide proper hair care at and early age, they will continue to strive for healthy hair care. This now young adult will wear styles that are becoming, styles that will enhance the young adult's beauty.

LOCATING PROFESSIONAL PRODUCTS FOR YOUR HAIR

These vary according to the texture of one's hair. Of course, all want to use products that give the most benefits and that is long lasting. Your hair professional should direct you in selecting the appropriate product for your hair. But, how do we adjust our budget while we desire to use a hair product that enhances the beauty of our hair and allow it to stay healthy. There are many ways to find these products at a discount price. Check on line for discount prices. Also, search out salons in your area that offer monthly discounts for professional hair products. You know that dollar discount store in your neighbor? Check them out too. They receive professional products from time to time, and there is always your local beauty supply store. If you can find your professional product at your local thrift store, why not go there, too? Remember, changing your products provides a different menu for your hair so don't be afraid to try something new, but be sure to read your labels. They often contain the information you need to ensure that a hair product will work well for you. Don't feel ashamed, healthy hair is your goal. If the price is right stock up for when your money is acting funny.

WHEN GROWING OUT YOUR RELAXER

Many are looking for relief on their pocketbook and they are realizing that there is beauty in their own natural hair. Some choose the extreme method of cutting their hair off completely. This is not necessary when growing out a relaxer. Allow your hair to grow out to a comfortable length that you can deal with. The line of demarcation will be evident. Moisturize, shampoo and use a deep conditioner with a hot oil treatment (use a disposable plastic cap as this will generate some heat). The allotted time should be fifteen minutes. These treatments should be done weekly. This will help your hair remain soft and manageable. Avoid brushing your hair when wet. Use a wide tooth comb to clear the hair out. Do not tug or pull on your hair, but comb it gently. There will be some hair breakage and hair loss during this process. The new hair growth texture is now different from the relaxed hair (this includes hair process with color and bleach,) this may cause the hair to snap. Once you have reach a comfortable length, it is time to have a professional haircut. Continue treatments is advised. Love it and wear it!

GOING NATURAL

There are many ways to wear your natural or curly hair. Some like to believe that their hair is (*nappy*), but it is just extremely curly. The best way to wear your natural hair is with respect and dignity. There are extremely tight curls, medium curls and long wavy curls. The texture defines the curl. The professional hair product you choose defines your curl. There is much variety when it comes to the diversity of natural hair what may work well for you may not for someone else. So keep an open mind, it's all beauty. Start your new look with a fresh haircut. Natural hair cuts better when it is dry, so why not blow dry it before cutting. There is much beauty in wearing your natural hair. Twisting and molding it into various styles on any day (not just on special occasions) adds genuine beauty. When searching out professional hair products, it may take time to find out what works best for your hair. Daily leave-in conditioner that will lock your curl into place accentuates beauty. Deep condition your hair to prevent dryness. Some find that Shea butter or hair wax helps to define their curls; others use oils of various kinds. These oils is not the same as a hair sheen or gloss that adds vibrancy to your look.

PERMANENT WAVE
AND YOUR HAIR

I enjoy rolling those bone rods; it was so easy. From straight hair to wavy curl hair (*the permanent wave chemical is not to be confused with the Curl or relaxer chemical mentioned on the previous pages*), there are more innovating techniques used for rolling long hair today which are great. The permanent wave curl can be very enhancing to those who do not want to spend thirty or sixty minutes each day doing their hair. It is a "wash and go" hair style. Others use it to build body to their hair. The permanent wave should make your hair look like a nice natural looking wave curl, not a muffin top *(get the picture?)*. A curl lock leave in conditioner define the curls. Alternating rod size gives a better flow. As a hair professional, I avoided doing perms on hair that is bleached. This double process is very damaging. A hair rinse is suitable for hair that is gray. There is wisdom founded when talking with those little old ladies that demand your attention when doing a permanent wave on their hair; some are quite funny. I learn a lot from them, so don't push them aside. Talk with them and they will be your client for life. That is unless they have a family member that is willing do their perms. Our economy has changed the way people think. Always seek a hair professional for this service. Their professional techniques give better results.

HAIR DECOR ORNAMENTS

Hair decorative ornaments of various kinds enhance the beauty of a hairstyle and are useful tools for special occasions. Please, be alert when using these hair decors to enhance the beauty of your hair. Avoid ones that cause breakage and remove these hair decors properly. It is recommend not to sleep with them in your hair. When using rubber bands for holding a hairstyle in place try doing so without it being too tight. When removing, snip clip with the tip of a pair of pointed scissors. Avoid pulling, breaking and snapping the hair. (I have observed some children's hair and skin pulled to tight; it looks painful.) When using them on children's hair, make sure the children are comfortable. Most children don't like to have their hair groomed because it hurts them, so be careful of their feelings make hair care enjoyable. Help them to see the beauty in it all.

HATS AND YOUR HAIR

Hats are like the wigs. You have to have one in your closet for a bad hair day. This can be very comfortable. Hats may define a mood, how we are feeling for the day. It can add attractiveness to and outfit or protect your hair from the sun, or it is just being you or whatever the case may be. Hats should be for personal use only. This aids in protecting your hair from unwanted bacteria. Sweat and bacteria builds up on the inside perimeter of hats, so cleaning your head wear on a regular basis is wise. Switch it up from time to time. Wear a silk scarf under your hat to avoid hair breakage if possible. Style may be important to you, but prolong use of hats can cause hair loss. Watch where you place your hat and place it opposite from the correct position for wearing. You know, upside down when resting it on an object. Never place it on the floor. We don't think about these things but bacteria is everywhere and can be carry to your hair and scalp.

WHERE YOU REST YOUR HEAD

Think about it where did you rest your head today. Was it in the doctor office against the wall while waiting to be seen for an appointment? Perhaps in a hospital emergency waiting room? Against the wall in the employees lounge, or just in the grass? Most people stretch their bodies out and rest their head backwards it comes natural. How many other persons did the same thing that day in the same spot? What about where pets play or sleep? How about when we see children rub their heads on the floor of your home or into the carpet. Think of the how much traffic goes back and forth. Now, think of the bacteria found in these areas. It may seem odd to mention this. This is food for thought. It is not to say that every where we lay our heads can cause us a problem with our hair or causes us to pick up bacteria. Some people may be more sensitive to bacteria than others. If this is the case, where you rest your hair does matter.

MENOPAUSE AND YOUR HAIR

One day, I walked into my salon to begin a day of work and my daughter said to me, "Mom, did you take your pill today?" I must have looked like I was losing my mind, but somehow, I thought I had it all together. This may be the most difficult time for a women and her hair. Some experience thinning and hair loss among other things.

Not all women are affected by this period in their life. When those hormones begin to change your life, it is best to use something to help control your hair loss. This is personal. You can discuss this with your doctor. Choose a hormone replacement therapy that works for you and your hair. Some prefer a more natural form of therapy. Whatever the case, if menopause is affecting your hair, do something about it. Refrain from using hair chemicals. If you are taking prescribed medication, remember to use hair products that cleanse and condition the hair so that it can remain as healthy as possible. A hair rinse works best if you cannot tolerate the grey. Semi-colors give the grey a highlighted look and tends to be less damaging. Look great, feel good and keep it in control.

THE GOLDEN HAIR

Shame is not for me. It brought the best out of me. My hair is not what it used to be, and I feel that I don't want you to see what it has done to me. I am surely happy in whatever I want my hair to be. No hair is fine for me if this is the way it has to be. IT'S ONLY TEMPORARY, you see. They make enough of it for me. So, the only thing that matters to me is the Golden YEARS!! I have come to see. So, I can adjust my life to whatever changing hair experience that suits me.—

~~*Detrice Milliner-Sims*

HUMAN PEOPLE
WITH HUMAN HAIR

Let's meet the world. Let's travel abroad and what do you find? People with human hair: Soft hair, fine hair, coarse hair, curly hair, straight hair, long hair, medium length hair, short hair, weary hair, cotton hair, hard hair, colorful hair, flyaway hair, spike hair, thin hair, thick hair, no hair, exotic hair, strong hair and weak hair. Did I miss one? If so, place it here: _____ hair.

Sandy's Hair

My culture is Indian and Spanish. I am from the country of Belize. My hair has much diversity. It's long and soft, silky and shiny. When I lived in Belize, a hair cream worked best for me. After moving to Los Angeles, California, I noticed that a change of climate left my hair spongy and curly. I had to use a different professional hair cream product. This helped my hair return to its naturalness. Now, I am living in Las Vegas and my hair has become dry in texture. I find that I have to wash it more frequently. I am still using a professional hair cream. While it is wet, I add a hair mousse that helps it to straighten. I wrap it around my head. This allows me to wear it in a nice style. Coloring and highlighting my hair adds to its attractiveness. I cannot, however, use hair relaxers on my hair because it literally melts it and it feels like wax.

Michelle is from Germany

I was over processing my hair with color when I met Dee, my hair professional. You see, my hair was blonde in color and I didn't want my grey to show, so I change it to red, but I was coloring it to soon each month. Now, my hair is thin. My hair professional was truthful. She helped me to understand that I had to make adjustments in the way I care for my hair. I did. It's still red. You see, I like that color. I think it makes me look sexy for my husband. Now, with proper hair care, I see a difference in its texture. It has thickened up a little. I have my hair cut in a flattering short and layered style. I always get nice comments. I have a hairstylist I can trust.

Casandra was born in El Paso, Texas

My mom is from Germany and my dad is from Alabama. My hair used to be lame and boring, just curly and hard to maintain, until I met my hairstylist. She educated me on how to care for my hair. Now, I have hair that has life. She cuts my hair so perfectly and in a nice style. She's taught me how to care for my hair and how to manage it. Twice a year, she gives me highlights. She said this is enough for a young teenager. Those highlights grow out so beautifully and allow my hair to stay healthy. She reminds me to apply hair oil and use shampoo and conditioner for color treated hair. She knows exactly what I want done and what I need. I don't have to worry that she will do the wrong thing. I will always go to her.

Arnett's Hair

In my youth, my hair was precious to me. It was shiny, thick and long. I felt good, it looked good and it was a wonderful way to change my looks. Our hair was very special to those who came from Sharpsburg, North Carolina. We work in the field during those heated summers and fall weather. The dirt and dust required us to wash our hair every weekend. We braided it or straightened it with a hot comb. Today, they call them flat irons. We always cut it and sometimes, we relaxed it, or did whatever made us feel beautiful. In my twenties and thirties it became a special way I pamper myself. I transformed myself, depending, on the outfit I was wearing or according to the times.

A job interview and a date were most important to me. Oh, how beautiful I felt when my hair was the way I wanted it to be. It built self-esteem and confidence and made me feel that I looked good in my outfits. Now those years have caught up with me and health issues have taken its toll, but guess what, I still have hair. What was once a joy is no more. For me to come close to feeling pretty, I have to wash it and use moisturizing conditioner. For now, I have a very short curly hair style with thinness taking over the sides and top of my head. How I miss the days of being a chameleon, remembering when I could change my looks just as I changed my wardrobe. I am in my fifties only hoping that my hair returns to the shine and style of what it used to be. As I approach my sixties, I long for the day when my hair and health would be like those days when I lived in Honolulu, Hawaii.

Terriah's Weave Nightmare (The Bobby Pin Fiasco)

For me, hair is a way of expressing a style, conveying a mood or hiding a flaw. There is beauty in it all. Booth good and traumatic experiences have shaped my view of hair and have only served as a means of furthering my curiosity, exploration and its experimentations of different forms. As I recall, several of my peers had this popular hairstyle of the times. I begged my mom to allow me to get a weave piece. Each time, she said, "No, why do you want a weave piece? You already have so much hair." I explained that my natural hair is not curly. One summer away from home, I convinced my sister to allow me to get that weave piece. I was so excited. "My first weave!" I will never forget that hairstyle, a curly-weave ponytail with twisties in the front. The beautician asked if I liked the way it looked. I responded, "Yes very much, but is it really supposed to be this tight?" She reassured me by saying, "Yes, don't worry it will loosen in a couple days." The first day I bopped around with so much confidence and no one could tell me I didn't look good. That same night, I developed a slight headache. My sister gave me an aspirin and said it was because I had never worn my hair like that before.

The next day, I woke up still with a lingering headache. That day I attended an event but the entire time I could not focus. That headache that was a number three was now a number nine. The following evening, I had reached my breaking point. I could not focus. I could not sleep. So, there I was with scissors in my hand and my sister assisting me. I carefully cut through that ponytail and my sister helped me unwrap it. She exclaimed in a large voice, "There's a bobby pin stuck in your scalp!" I was in disbelief! I ran to the mirror and it was wedged deep into my scalp and it was bleeding. With proper sanitation, I had my sister painfully remove it from my scalp. From that moment I promised myself I would never weave my hair again. To this day, that part of my head is still tender. It was several years before I would even reconsider the idea of weaving my hair again. Now, twenty-six years of age, the thing that I had once feared and denounced is now a regular fixture in my life.

My exploration continued and I found different textures, designs, hair braiding and coloring along with hair weaving to be a joy and a convenience I love. Whether I'm rocking my own natural hair or a fresh weave, I am always me.

Lin's Hair

My experience with hair has been a bit like a roller coaster filled with ups and downs, highs and lows. Memories of mom pressing and tying my hair up into a ponytail with ribbons sit so vividly in my mind. Words cannot even fathom the feeling of how each year I worked so hard to assist in the growth progress; and every year watching it grow and then fall out. At the age of nine, the doctor informed my mother I would continue to face this harsh reality of losing my hair every year as a result of Scarlet Fever. I had contracted it from a close neighborhood friend. By the same token, I was also informed that because of the severity of my condition, I would possibly be unable to have children. One year, I had embarked on a regimen of using specially formulated hair grease and the results were outstanding. For the first time, since I was a young child, my hair had grown past my shoulders and appeared to be full and healthy. Regrettably, later the following year and after relocation, I noticed shedding on a grand scale. Within a short time, I was back at my starting point. I have since made peace with this reality. I have over the years tried many hairstyles.

I have tried wearing Afros, short-lined Naturals, finger wave, press and curls, lined up fades, weaves, braids, pineapples curl, being bald and wigs. I never let my hair define me but only at times, define a mood. Though each year the strands may fall, I am thankful when I look at the smiling faces of my children and their children and remember the doctor was only right about one thing.

Dunnetta's Hair

My natural hair color is dark brown, but now I have grey hair on the top front part of my head. I like to use color to hide my gray, Red and Oriental Black is my favorite. I have long hair past my shoulders. The texture of my hair is coarse and fine with a wavy curl. I like to twist my natural hair sometimes. Many seem to compliment me when I wear it this way. I also like to where it in a ponytail style. I use a professional hair product that leaves it manageable so I can blow dry it and straighten it with a hot comb and or use a flat iron to get the look I want. I have a trusted member of my family who is a hair professional. She cuts and cares for my hair. I love you, baby sister. Thanks for being a good and trusted hairstylist.

Earthell's Hair Color

Having my hair color is a mood-enhancing experience. It makes me feel better about myself. It takes years off my looks. My husband also feels better when I color my hair because he doesn't like the grey. I always get nice comments when the color compliments my facial complexion and when it blends nicely with my highlights. It looks attractive. It grabs the attention of other females who say how nice it looks.

Felishia

My hairstylist is like the part of the family!!! I call her grandma. She taught me how to care for my hair! Before, I used to freak out whenever I would go to get my haircut the hairstylist always cut too much. But my hairstylist understands what I mean when I say, "Just a trim." (*Hahahaha*). She would try different colors sometimes and I would love each one. She take the time to find out what I really want. Yes, she's taught me how to love my hair in its different forms (I *love* her!!!).

Rosie's Hair

My mom is from Mexico City and my dad is from Arkansas. My natural hair color was dark brown, yet it is not coarse. It is soft and light. I have had many, MANY types of hair styles and colors. I've been a redhead, a brunette, a blonde and have had colors in between, such as burgundy and Kool-Aid red. I even let my hair grow out to its natural color. I'm 56 years old so that pretty much means it is salt and peppery grey. Over the years, however, I have had hair styles "of the day." I've used hair straighteners and permanents many times. I have damaged my hair because I didn't want to spend the time and money on hair stylists. I figured I could do the job just as well as any hairstylist. After all, I could read the directions on the box, right? Wrong! So wrong. I could read the directions, but I could not perform the task the way a professional hair stylist does. I finally met Dee. She is now my hair stylist. She currently cares for my hair. She educates me on how to care for my hair to keep my hair healthy. What I have learned from her in keeping my hair healthy has helped me to look and feel good. If my hair doesn't look good, I don't look good. If it looks tired, I look tired. Needless to say, I look and feel good all the time now. Thank you, Dee!

John's Hair ("The Long and Short of It.")

In high school (in the 60s), most of the "good" kids had crew cuts or just short hair. I graduated from high school in 1962 and I had long hair. Did this mean I was not a "good" kid? Well, I was not an angel, but I did not get into trouble.

When I joined the Army, I HAD to get a buzz cut, but I still managed to have more hair than others after basic training. While in the army, every inspection was the same, "You are border-line with that hair, Rios!" and I had just gotten a haircut that day!

After the army, I had a government job for 30 years and I wore my hair short. I grew out my hair long into a ponytail just before I retired from my job. I always cared for my hair by using professional hair products and by visiting my hair stylist once a month for a hair trim. I attribute the health of my hair to proper hair care.

Nash's Hair ("Healthy Scalp")

My wife cuts my "peach fuzz." I shampoo and condition my scalp with conditioning skin anti-septic, then give it a shine. My scalp looks so healthy and everyone says I wear it well.

Danay's Hair

"Not one [sparrow] will fall to the ground without your Father's knowledge. But the very hairs of your head are all numbered."—MATTHEW 10:29, 30. It is with this scripture that I begin because even our God cares about our hair!! Very comforting.

My overall experience with my hair has been … frustrating!! Primarily because I never really like to get my hair done (takes too long). I prefer to do it myself! I also don't like to spend a lot of money to get it done, and we all know the old adages: "you get what you pay for" . . . so sometimes saving money has turned out good for me, and other times I have deeply regretted it!

I can say I have tried many, many different things with my hair. Highlights, dyes, natural dyes, deep conditioning, mask, natural conditioners . . . . the list goes on. I have been many colors of the rainbow from dark, dark brown to light, light blonde. I have had all different lengths and styles (gotta switch it up, ya know?) from super long down my back to short above my shoulders, layers, bobs, and bangs. My favorite so far has been when my hair is light brown with a few blonde highlights and medium-length.

I started to have my hair "highlighted" at age 18 and have never looked back. My only knowledge of my true natural color is from pictures (kind of sad huh).

I also take after my mom so my hair is on the finer side, so I have tried many thickening agents. Living in Las Vegas, it is hard to keep hair from getting dry because it is simply so dry here! So many conditioners and masks are necessary.

Janelle's New Look

I am a twelve years old. My mom made a hair appointment for me to receive a keratin relaxing treatment. To maintain the healthiness of my hair and to keep the keratin in place, I had to follow specific instructions. For the first seventy-two hours, I could not wash my hair. I also had to use a straightener to adhere to the keratin. The following three things were important so that my hair could remain healthy:

> The use of a sulfate-free shampoo
> A conditioner that contains keratin ingredients
> Wear a swimming cap to protect my hair from any chemicals
> use in the pool

Virginia's Hair

I shampoo and condition my hair once a week. I give the ends special conditioning treatments because they are always very dry. The medication I take and the chemicals found in our water supply turn it yellow. So, to keep it white, I use a concentrated bluing non-toxic, biodegradable hair rinse. After rinsing, I apply castor oil, then comb and brush it. This helps it maintain the shine and keeps it healthy. I use a protein styling gel. On special occasions, I press it and curl it with hair rollers. Knowing how to care for my hair has kept it healthy.

Amir

I would like to tell you how I like and don't like the barbershop so much. First, I like the barbershop when I'm done because I look good after, and I like the booster seat that I have to sit on when I'm getting my hair cut. That's two things that I like about the barbershop. Sometimes, I don't like the barbershop because it hurts when I'm getting my hair cut. By-the-way, my dad is a barber. *He* cuts my hair."

Denita

I think that the best thing about my hair experience is that after all this time I feel I've come full circle. From my teen years during the 70's, when I first wore my hair "natural," to the many varied looks in between. I am now wearing an afro again.

I was actually in my early twenties before I began using chemicals to change my hair. At first, I started with a texturizer, which loosened the curl pattern just enough to make my hair more manageable

Next, I decided to try the Jeri Curl, and I loved that look for several years. When I started to get bored with that look, I had my hair colored a couple of times, just for something new.

When I really wanted a different look, I started buying wigs so that I could totally change my hairstyle. Finally, I tried a relaxer. I wore my hair in a variety of long and short styles through the years, but the wildest "do" I ever tried was the "Pineapple Wave," so named because of the lines and shape that the hair is put into by using a sculpting gel that hardens to the touch. Once it hardens, I bet even hurricane force winds couldn't move the hair around! Needless to say, I never tried that again.

Because my hair started breaking off, I eventually had to take a break from relaxers, and I started wearing tie-knots. After about a year, I decided to try a weave for the first time, and I went back to the relaxer for a while.

Then, I decided to try micro-braids and was referred to someone else. I wore my hair braided for about six months, and later, I decided to stop with the chemicals for good.

I switched back and forth between wearing wigs, weaves and tie-knots for a couple of years. During this time, I met Detrice, who helped me by styling one of my wigs as well as my weaves a few times. She gave me great advice about some wonderful hair products to use as well as giving me a fantastic hair cut that looked fresh and natural! Over the past several months, I have decided to try wearing my hair natural once in a while, so now I've been alternating that with wearing wigs again, and I love it! I sometimes twist my hair and leave it, or gently finger-comb it so that it's crinkly and wavy. Either way, I enjoy not having to worry about my hair. Who knows when it will be time for another change, but they say "variety is the spice of life," and I like things spicy!

Detrice Milliner-Sims

This was the most uncomfortable experience in my life. I received a chemical relaxer and my scalp began to burn. Needless to say, it had to be removed quickly. In the weeks to come, I found myself in the hospital. The doctor said that I had a tumor that could not be removed. They told my husband to prepare for my funeral. How devastating this was to me.

I later was informed that it was not a tumor. I had contracted Impetigo (a skin infection, with small blisters filled with fluid and when burst, formed a yellow-like crust.) The doctor ordered my hair to be shaved off. I sat and watched it just fall to the floor. The doctor's order was to clean my head with peroxide. It felt better. The infection continued to ooze. There were several interns that visited me in the course of my hospital stay. They were very kind in following the doctor orders; but, there was a female intern who new what I was dealing with. You see, once a day was not enough to clean and treat this infection. It needed to be done three times a day. I had to use a brush to scrub my scalp with an anti-bacteria cleanser while bursting the blister. The Impetigo was feeding on the moisture on my head. It was spreading to the other hair follicles. I remained in the hospital for two weeks and was treated with antibiotics. After leaving the hospital, I continued this treatment and daily applied an anti-bacteria ointment to the infected area. It took one year with medication to treat this infection.

A daily routine of bleaching and cleaning the towel that I used on my pillow each night killed the bacteria. My hair began to grow. How happy I was. The section of the hair where the infection began had destroyed those hair follicles. I had to wear hats for a while. In the privacy of my home, I allowed my scalp to get air which helped tremendously. With three inches of hair growth, I cut my hair into a short sassy hairstyle. I received many compliments. I embrace my natural hair. For a different look, I color and flat iron it and enjoy wearing braids during the summer months. Both my scalp and my hair are very healthy.

HAIR

Healthy • Acceptance • Inspiring • Reality

I LIKE YOU NOW AND I LIKE YOU THEN.

I LIKE YOU, THE WAY YOU SMILE, SO PLEASE DO IT AGAIN.

YOUR *HAIR* AND SKIN, HOW COLORFUL IT IS TO ME.

IT'S SMOOTH AND SOFT, THE WAY IT SUPPOSED TO BE.

THE HUGS OF LOVE, THIS IS WHAT I SEE.

I LIKE YOU NOW AND LIKE YOU THEN.

YOU'RE SO DIFFERENT. YOU ARE MY FRIEND.

WHO ARE YOU? WHERE DID YOU COME FROM?

I WANT TO KNOW WHY, AND I WANT TO KNOW HOW

AND I WANT TO KNOW WHEN. PLEASE, PLEASE TELL ME . . . WOW!

LET'S DO IT AGAIN AND AGAIN.

PEOPLE, YOUR *HAIR* IS YOUR FRIEND.

~~*DETRICE MILLINER-SIMS*

A PASSION TO SHARE

It's all hair secrets some may think. The truth is there are no secrets. Attending cosmetology school taught me how to work in the hair profession. It was a time when if you graduated from high school, you could get a good job. Suddenly, that changed because now, a college degree is needed.

So, I went to college only to find out that it was not for me. Secretarial, medical and nursing courses gave me the ability to find and hold a job, but that was it. My heart was in the business of hair. I enjoyed the leg work; being a sharer and a giver to please the best I could. I enjoyed the people contact and the challenge to create while it define my personality. I realized and understood life changes and how to make adjustments, when needed. There were no secrets. I just enjoyed what I was doing.

Now, I can share my experience with others. Knowledge is for sharing. This helps us to feel complete, so why not share my developed passion for the field of hair? What I share can benefit others. Everyone wants to tell a story. I just wanted to share my experiences because that what makes a life story. That passion I developed for hair is for sharing now. Sharing what we know gives meaning to life.

A MEMO TO HAIR PROFESSIONALS

As a hair professional, I met many challenges and my share of mistakes. There is one thing I have learned and that is to respect yourself, respect your clients and have them respect you.

If you are an honest hairstylist, you will draw honest people. If you are a flakey hairstylist, you will draw flakey people. If your salon is a hangout joint, you will draw those kinds of clients. You set the tone for your business and your clients.

Plan your future well and plan for the day you retire. While you are making those big bucks, why not invest it into a retirement plan or perhaps report that income and tips to the IRS. My fellow hairstylists laughed at me when I was doing that. Paying my taxes over the years now provides me with an income to maintain my self-respect.

www.ingramcontent.com/pod-product-compliance
Lightning Source LLC
Chambersburg PA
CBHW020400290526
45785CB00005B/2384